LEUKEMIA DIET PLAN HANBOOK

How to Eat and Stay
Healthy While Fighting
Leukemia

DR. ANDREW STOREY

Table of Contents

CHAPTER ONE

Eating a diet for leukemia

How to Eat and Stay Healthy
While Fighting Leukemia

Nutrition, along with rest and exercise, is critical in the fight against leukemia. During and after treatment for leukemia, it is important to eat a diet that supports a healthy body and immune system. Leukemia and its treatments can have a number of side effects that necessitate specialized nutrition advice.

In terms of healthy eating, guidelines for leukemia patients do not differ greatly from those for the general population. Dietary considerations for those with leukemia are outlined below. You may have additional health concerns, such as food allergies or gastrointestinal issues, that necessitate special consideration for these nutritional guidelines.

The spleen can grow in size as a side effect of some types of leukemia, and what you eat can either help or worsen this side effect. Before making major changes to your diet, always consult with your doctor.

Dietary Recommendations for People With Leukemia

It's a good idea to stick to a mostly plant-based diet, but you can include some meat and dairy products. A Mediterranean diet and a plant-based diet tend to go hand in hand. These foods include fruits, vegetables, whole grains, low-fat dairy, lean meats and other protein sources as well as healthy fats in the form of nuts and seeds. Reduce your daily calorie intake by no more than 10% if you want to avoid the dangers of saturated fats like those found in butter and fried foods.

Increasing your intake of antioxidants is one of the many benefits of a plant-based diet. Antioxidants protect against cancer-causing free radicals.

"My oncologist told me to try to stay on a Mediterranean diet for overall health. Another member admitted, "I eat mostly chicken, turkey, and fish." As for my daily diet, I eat a lot of fresh vegetables (kale, spinach, and collard greens), brown rice, and fruit as snacks. Drink a cup of tea or water. "Make an effort to increase your intake of vegetables."

Curcumin, Ursolic Acid, and Cruciferous Vegetables

Ursolic acid may be able to inhibit tumor growth by affecting mitochondrial function and metabolic pathways. Apples, basil, rosemary, and cranberries all contain ursolic acid. It's safe to cook with or eat these ingredients, but supplementing with them isn't recommended right now.

Glucosinolates, which are found in cruciferous vegetables, may help prevent and treat cancer. This compound has been shown in studies to help fight cancers of the lungs, colon, breast, and prostate. In order to better understand the health benefits of glucosinolates, additional research is needed. Broccoli, Brussels sprouts, and cauliflower are all examples of cruciferous vegetables, as are other similar crops.

The anticancer properties of curcumin are attributed to this compound. Different cell signaling pathways, including growth factors and cytokines, may be targeted by this treatment to help prevent or recurrence of cancer. Studies show that black pepper may improve the absorption of curcumin, which has a low bioavailability and is rapidly eliminated from the body. Preliminary clinical trials are needed to determine the efficacy of this compound.

While curcumin, cruciferous vegetables, and ursolic acid may not be directly linked to blood cancers, they contain immune-boosting compounds. These may aid in the fight against leukemia-related infections, a common complication of treatment.

CHAPTER TWO

Fiber

The importance of fiber in a healthy diet is often overlooked. Starchy foods like vegetables, fruits, whole grains, legumes, nuts, and seeds are rich in fiber, which can be found in these foods. Fiber aids digestion, lowers blood sugar, regulates lipids, and boosts the population of beneficial bacteria in the gut. Women need at least 25 grams of fiber per day, and men need at least 35 grams of fiber per day for optimal health.

"I never get constipated because I tend to 'overdose' on high-fiber foods. Fruits and vegetables, whole-wheat pasta and bread are some of the best options for weight loss.

A high-fiber diet may aggravate stomach discomfort and worsen nausea in some people dealing with leukemia. You may be advised by your doctor to follow a low-fiber diet in these situations.

Vitamin D is essential for a healthy immune system.

In order to move your muscles and send signals to your nerves, your body needs vitamin D. As well as your body's ability to fight off disease-causing bacteria and viruses, your immune system is also important. Additionally, vitamin D helps the body absorb calcium, which is essential for bone health.

Vitamin D intake and leukemia symptoms are not yet clearly linked, but some studies suggest that it may be beneficial. Other sources of vitamin D include salmon and sardines, some vegetables and legumes (like kale and soybeans), and fortified products such as milk, cereals, and orange juice.

Using a plate

A well-balanced diet is easier to achieve when using the plate method. Portion control and distribution are critical because even a good thing can be harmful in excess.

• Vegetables should make up half of your plate, and the more vibrant the better.

Protein, such as chicken, fish, or legumes, should comprise one-quarter of your plate.

Brown rice, quinoa, or sweet potato can make up a quarter of your meal.

An olive oil, avocado, or nut or seed based fat is an excellent addition to any meal. Protein and fiber in fruit can help manage blood sugar levels and make you feel more satisfied after eating it, whether as a meal or a snack. Pair apple slices with almond butter, grapes with string cheese, or bell pepper strips with hummus, for example. They all go well together.

You can indulge in your favorite foods in moderation as a part of a healthy meal distribution. It's better to indulge in a small amount of your favorite sweet rather than deprive yourself and risk overindulging later.

Eat whatever you want in moderation," a member advised. "Live in the now, because tomorrow is not guaranteed."

While Treating Leukemia, Maintaining a Healthy Weight

Weight management is essential to overall health. If you are overweight or obese, you should eat enough calories to maintain a healthy weight or to lose weight gradually.

Malnutrition can be difficult to avoid if you're experiencing nausea, vomiting, diarrhoea or other symptoms of food poisoning. During these times, it's critical to focus on foods that are high in calories and high in nutrients. Calorie intake and protein intake are both critical for weight management and maintaining lean muscle mass.

Choosing foods that are high in both nutrients and calories is a good idea if you or your doctor are concerned about weight loss during or after leukemia treatment. Consider these possible choices:

- Nuts

Peanut butter and other nut butters

- Avocados

- Beans

- Chicken

- Fish

- Yogurt

If you don't want to eat solid food, smoothies and soups are two popular options. Nutritional foods such as flaxseed, chia seeds, nut butters, beans, and vegetables can be easily disguised in soup and smoothies.

You can also get enough calories by eating more frequently or in smaller portions throughout the day rather than only one or two large meals. A healthy appetite can be stimulated by regular physical activity.

After making dietary adjustments, some MyLeukemiaTeam members reported weight loss and improved well-being. One member revealed, "I stopped eating sugar and processed food back in March." Aside from the fact that I've lost 30 pounds, I've felt a lot better since then.

Maintaining a healthy weight can also help with the management of potentially harmful weight-related health conditions. "I went four months without eating carbs or sugar." My diabetes and extremely fatty liver healed themselves. My doctor has been so pleased with my progress," another member of the group said.

CHAPTER THREE

Anemia, a condition brought on by a lack of red blood cells or iron, is common in people with leukemia. With proper nutrition, anemia may be alleviated. The iron intake of people with anemia must be monitored.

Both heme and nonheme iron are available. Animal sources such as meat, poultry, and fish contain heme iron that is only about 15% absorbed by the body. Iron from nonheme sources, like legumes and grains, can only be absorbed at a rate of 3 to 8 per cent. Several factors have the potential to influence iron absorption in either a positive or negative way.

It is a good rule of thumb to include some vitamin C in your diet at every meal, especially those that are rich in iron. Iron absorption in the body is improved by vitamin C. Ascorbic acid (Vitamin C) can be found in a wide variety of fruits and vegetables. Coffee and tea consumption has been shown to significantly reduce iron absorption. Drinking these beverages with meals that are high in iron is a bad idea.

Vitamin B12 and folic acid deficiency may cause megaloblastic anemia, a rare form of anemia. If you've been diagnosed with acute myeloid leukemia or myelodysplastic syndromes, you may develop megaloblastic anemia. Vitamin B12 and folic acid can be found in a wide variety of foods.

Top Vitamin B12 Sources:

• Clams

- Cereal with added nutrients

- Tuna

- Non-fat plain Greek yogurt.

- Salmon

- Beef

- Chicken

- Eggs

- Brewer's yeast

Top Folic Acid Sources:

- Spinach

- Cereal with added nutrients

- Black-eyed peas /

- Asparagus

- Brussel Sprouts, on the other hand, are

- Broccoli

- Avocado

Kidney Failure

Kidney damage is a side effect that can occur in people with leukemia. Your doctor may recommend a specific diet if your bloodwork shows signs of kidney damage. In some cases, it may be necessary to restrict potassium, sodium, and phosphorus-rich foods to treat kidney problems. The results of your blood tests will be monitored by your doctor to determine if you need to limit the intake of any of these nutrients. Then you might be asked to limit:

fruits and vegetables rich in potassium, such as citrus fruits and bananas

Dairy products such as cheese and bread as well as nuts and seeds high in phosphorus

Salty foods, such as salty snacks, condiments, salad dressings, sauces, and food served at restaurants and takeout establishments

Hydration

Nutritional transport, joint health, blood pressure

regulation, and so much more are all influenced by a person's water intake. Hydration with water is the most effective method. You should avoid sugary drinks like soda and fruit juice, or at least limit their consumption. Try adding fresh fruit, fruit extract, or low-sugar sports drinks such as G2 by Gatorade, Propel flavored electrolyte water, or Vitaminwater Zero if you're not a fan of plain water.

Women should have no more than one drink a day, and men should have no more than two.

As previously mentioned, plan your coffee and tea intake to avoid limiting your iron absorption.

"I drink V8 +Energy tea before workouts and swimming laps," said another member. Maybe it's just in my head, but it gives me the energy I need."

The Core Power drink has a lot of protein, according to one of our members. A 42-gram protein option is available. Once a day or so, I'll drink half a bottle."

People With Leukemia's Food Safety

People with leukemia, whose immune systems are weakened by the condition known as leukopenia, must pay special attention to food safety (low white blood cell count). The risk of foodborne illness is greater for stem cell transplant patients than for those who receive chemotherapy and radiation alone.

CHAPTER FOUR

To avoid contracting a foodborne illness, follow these simple dos and don'ts when handling food.

Observe the following guidelines to ensure the safety of your food:

• Be sure to thoroughly cook all meat and fish.

• Make sure the eggs are cooked all the way through.

Peeled produce should be thoroughly washed before

handling. Use an apple cider vinegar and water solution to kill bacteria on fruits and vegetables before eating.

Refrigerate all deli meats, even those that have been dry-cured.

Don'ts for Food Safety:.

Make your own mayonnaise or cookie dough and eat the raw eggs.

• Consume raw milk or juice.

• Consume soft cheeses like brie, blue cheese, and Gorgonzola. •

• Because food sits for longer periods of time, it is more likely to become contaminated, so stick to salad bars and buffets.

Make sure to eat a lot of alfalfa or other fresh sprouts.

In the absence of boiling or filtering, do not drink well water.

Nutritional and Supplement Facts to Consider

It can be difficult to sort through nutrition supplement and cancer health claims to determine what is true and what is merely a marketing gimmick. There is insufficient scientific evidence to support the use of a specific nutrient or supplement in cancer treatment.

Before taking any supplement or herb, you should always consult with your doctor. Your cancer treatment may suffer as a result. Imatinib (Gleevec), a drug used to treat chronic myeloid leukemia and Philadelphia-positive acute lymphoblastic leukemia, is known to be reduced in effectiveness by St. John's wort, a popular herbal supplement. Bortezomib, a chemotherapy drug used to treat multiple myeloma and mantle cell lymphoma, can also be affected by green tea supplements.

Each Person's Dietary Requirements Are Individual

Depending on how well you respond to leukemia treatment, additional nutrition advice must be tailored to your specific needs. chemotherapy and radiation have a wide range of side effects, including:

- Lack of desire to eat

Predictable satiety

- Nausea

- Vomiting

- Mouth dryness

Sores in the mouth

Changes or loss of taste in the mouth

- A hard time swallowing.

- Constipation

- Diarrhea

It is possible to alleviate these side effects by consulting with your doctor, a registered dietitian, or a nutritionist, who can help you maintain a healthy diet that will make you feel your best.

THE END